JUICING AND SMOOTHIES FOR ACNE

Quick and easy anti aging fruit juice to overcome acne and maintenance of your skin

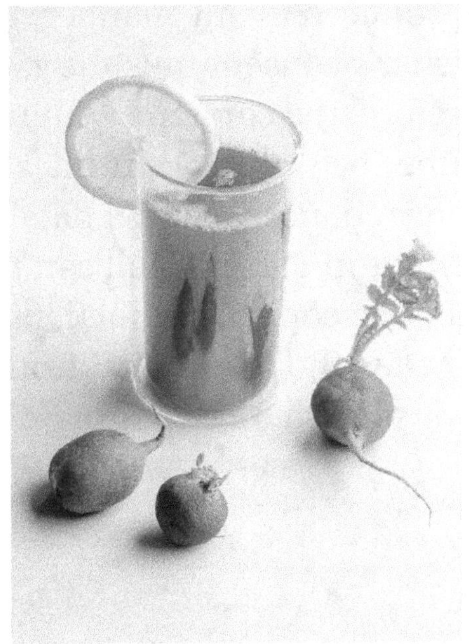

Dr. Malvin Harison

TABLE OF CONTENT

Introduction   3

The Significance of Taking the Right juice and
Smoothie   5

Chapter 1: 30 Juicing Recipes for acne   7

1. Green Goddess   7
2. Carrot Zinger   8
3. Berry Blast   8
4. Citrus Refresher   9
5. Pineapple Paradise   10
6. Veggie Delight   11
7. Tropical Twist   12
8. Cucumber Cooler   13
9. Beet Blast   13
10. Apple Delight   14
11. Kale Kick   15
12. Watermelon Wonder   17
13. Healing Turmeric   17
14. Spinach Supreme   18
15. Papaya Paradise   19
16. Ginger Lemonade   20
17. Mango Madness   21
18. Raspberry Refresher   22
19. Carrot Glow   22
20. Pomegranate Punch   23
21. Citrus Sunrise   24
22. Green Detox   25
23. Minty Melon   27
24. Beet Blast   28

25. Berry Beet Bliss 29

26. Citrus Ginger Zing 30

27. Kiwi Lime Cooler 31

28. Creamy Avocado Delight 31

29. Ginger Turmeric Elixir 33

30. Creamy Green 34

Chapter 2: 30 delicious Smoothie Recipes for acne 35

1. Green Glow Smoothie 35

2. Berry Burst Smoothie 35

3. Citrus Zing Smoothie 36

4. Tropical Delight Smoothie 36

5. Glow-Getter Smoothie 37

6. Avocado Elixir Smoothie 37

7. Blueberry Bliss Smoothie 38

8. Minty Melon Smoothie 38

9. Pineapple Paradise Smoothie 39

10. Super Berry Blast Smoothie 39

11. Creamy Green Dream Smoothie 40

12. Chocolate Bliss Smoothie 40

13. Golden Sunshine Smoothie 41

14. Matcha Magic Smoothie 42

15. Protein Powerhouse Smoothie 42

16. Zen Garden Smoothie 43

17. Lavender Dream Smoothie: 43

18. Exotic Dragon Smoothie 44

19. Chia Power Smoothie 45

20. Mocha Madness Smoothie: 45

21. Enchanted Forest Smoothie 46

22. Cosmic Galaxy Smoothie: 46

23. Rainbow Bliss Smoothie 47

24. Unicorn Sparkle Smoothie 48

25. Mermaid's Delight Smoothie 48

26. Phoenix Rising Smoothie 49

27. Fairy Dust Smoothie 50

28. Centaur's Strength Smoothie 50

29. Time Traveler's Elixir Smoothie 51

30. Galaxy Explorer Smoothie: 52

Chapter 3:Bonus **53**

21 tips to reduce acne 53

Conclusion **58**

Introduction

Welcome to "Acne Juicing and Smoothies for Beginners" – your ultimate guide to unlocking radiant skin through the art of blending. Bid farewell to conventional skincare and embark on a journey where vibrant fruits, nutrient-packed veggies, and superfoods unite to create delicious elixirs designed to transform your complexion from the inside out.

Whether you're a juicing novice or a blending maestro, our carefully crafted recipes cater to all levels of expertise. Get ready to sip your way to clearer skin and embrace the transformative power of nature's goodness. Your journey to a blemish-free glow begins here. Cheers to a healthier, more radiant you!

The Significance of Taking the Right juice and Smoothie

In the quest for clearer skin, the significance of choosing the right juice and smoothie recipes cannot be overstated. Beyond being a mere trend, the careful selection of ingredients in these concoctions holds the key to addressing acne at its root.

The synergy of nutrient-packed fruits, vegetables, and superfoods in these recipes goes beyond mere taste – it's a strategic approach to nourishing your body from within. By incorporating ingredients rich in antioxidants, vitamins, and minerals known for their skin-loving properties, you're providing your body with the tools it needs to combat inflammation, support collagen production, and promote overall skin health.

Moreover, the simplicity and convenience of juicing and smoothies make them an accessible and enjoyable part of your daily routine. They effortlessly integrate into busy lifestyles, offering a tasty solution for those seeking an effective and holistic approach to skincare.

1. Green Goddess

Ingredients:
- 2 cups spinach
- 1 cucumber
- 2 celery stalks
- 1 green apple
- 1 lemon (juiced)

Instructions:
1. Wash all the ingredients thoroughly.
2. Cut the cucumber, celery, and green apple into smaller pieces.
3. Add all the ingredients to a juicer and extract the juice.
4. Stir well and serve immediately.

Serving Size: 1 glass
Nutritional Value: Rich in vitamins A, C, and K, and antioxidants.
Cooking Time: 5 minutes

2. Carrot Zinger

Ingredients:
- 4 carrots
- 1-inch piece of ginger
- 1 orange (peeled)

Instructions:
1. Wash and peel the carrots and ginger.
2. Chop them into small pieces.
3. Peel the orange and separate it into segments.
4. Put all the ingredients into a juicer and extract the juice.
5. Mix well and serve chilled.

Serving Size: 1 glass
Nutritional Value: High in vitamin A, C, and antioxidants.
Cooking Time: 5 minutes

3. Berry Blast

Ingredients:
- 1 cup strawberries
- 1 cup blueberries
- 1 cup raspberries
- 1 cup blackberries
- 1 tablespoon honey (optional)

Instructions:
1. Wash all the berries thoroughly.
2. Add the berries to a juicer and extract the juice.
3. Sweeten with honey if desired.
4. Stir well and serve over ice.
Serving Size: 1 glass
Nutritional Values: Packed with antioxidants with vitamin C.
Cooking Time: 5 minutes

4. Citrus Refresher

Ingredients:
- 2 oranges (peeled)
- 1 grapefruit (peeled)
- 1 lime (juiced)
- 1 tablespoon honey (optional)

Instructions:
1. Peel the oranges and grapefruit, and separate them into segments.
2. Juice the lime.
3. Add the citrus fruits and lime juice to a juicer and extract the juice.
4. Sweeten with honey if desired.
5. Stir well and serve chilled.

Serving Size: 1 glass
Nutritional Value: Rich in vitamin C and antioxidants.
Cooking Time: 5 minutes

5. Pineapple Paradise

Ingredients:
- 2 cups fresh pineapple chunks
- 1 cucumber
- 1 handful fresh mint leaves
- 1 lemon (juiced)

Instructions:
1. Wash the cucumber and mint leaves.
2. Chop the cucumber into small pieces.
3. Add the pineapple chunks, cucumber, mint leaves, and lemon juice to a juicer and extract the juice.
4. Mix well and serve over ice.

Serving Size: 1 glass
Nutritional Value: Contains bromelain, vitamin C, and antioxidants.
Cooking Time: 5 minutes

6. Veggie Delight

Ingredients:
- 2 carrots
- 2 tomatoes
- 1 beetroot
- 1 handful spinach
- 1-inch piece of ginger
- 1 lemon (juiced)

Instructions:
1. Wash the carrots, tomatoes, beetroot, and spinach.
2. Peel the carrots and beetroot and chop them into small pieces.
3. Chop the tomatoes into quarters.
4. Peel the ginger.
5. Add all the ingredients to a juicer and extract the juice.
6. Stir well and serve chilled.

Serving Size: 1 glass

Nutritional Value: Rich in vitamins A, C, and antioxidants.

Cooking Time: 7 minutes

7. Tropical Twist

Ingredients:
- 1 mango (peeled and pitted)
- 1 cup pineapple chunks
- 1 orange (peeled)
- 1 banana

Instructions:
1. Peel and chop the mango, pineapple, and orange.
2. Peel the banana and cut it into chunks.
3. Add all the ingredients to a blender and blend until smooth.
4. Serve over ice.

Serving Size: 1 glass

Nutritional Value: Contains vitamin C, beta-carotene, and fiber.

Cooking Time: 5 minutes

8. Cucumber Cooler

Ingredients:
- 2 cucumbers
- 1 cup fresh mint leaves
- 1 lime (juiced)
- 1 tablespoon honey (optional)

Instructions:

1. Wash the cucumbers and mint leaves.

2. Chop the cucumbers into small pieces.

3. Add the cucumber pieces, mint leaves, and lime juice to a blender and blend until smooth.

4. Sweeten with honey if desired.

5. Serve chilled.

Serving Size: 1 glass

Nutritional Value: Hydrating and rich in vitamins and minerals.

Cooking Time: 5 minutes

9. Beet Blast

Ingredients:

- 2 beetroots
- 2 carrots
- 1 apple
- 1 lemon (juiced)

Instructions:

1. Wash and peel the beetroots, carrots, and apples.

2. Chop them into small pieces.

3. Add the beetroot, carrot, apple, and lemon juice to a juicer and extract the juice.

4. Stir well and serve immediately.

Serving Size: 1 glass

Nutritional Value: Rich in antioxidants, vitamins A, C, and iron.

Cooking Time: 5 minutes

10. Apple Delight

Ingredients:

- 4 apples
- 1-inch piece of ginger
- 1 lemon (juiced)

Instructions:

1. Wash and chop the apples into small pieces.

2. Peel the ginger.

3. Add the apple pieces, ginger, and lemon juice to a juicer and extract the juice.

4. Stir well and serve chilled.

Serving Size: 1 glass

Nutritional Value: High in antioxidants, vitamin C, and fiber.

Cooking Time: 5 minutes

11. Kale Kick

Ingredients:
- 2 cups kale leaves
- 2 green apples
- 1 cucumber
- 1 lemon (juiced)

Instructions:
1. Wash the kale leaves and cucumber.
2. Chop the kale leaves, green apples, and cucumber into small pieces.
3. Add all the ingredients to a juicer and extract the juice.
4. Mix well and serve over ice.

Serving Size: 1 glass
Nutritional Value: Rich in vitamins A, C, and K, and antioxidants.
Cooking Time: 5 minutes

12. Watermelon Wonder

Ingredients:
- 2 cups watermelon chunks
- 1 lime (juiced)
- 1 handful fresh mint leaves

Instructions:
1. Remove the seeds from the watermelon chunks.
2. Add the watermelon chunks, lime juice, and mint leaves to a blender and blend until smooth.
3. Serve chilled.
Serving Size: 1 glass
Nutritional Value: Hydrating and rich in vitamin C and antioxidants.
Cooking Time: 5 minutes

13. Healing Turmeric

Ingredients:
- 1 large carrot
- 1 orange (peeled)
- 1-inch piece of turmeric root
- 1 lemon (juiced)

Instructions:

1. Wash and peel the carrot and orange.
2. Chop them into small pieces.
3. Peel the turmeric root.
4. Add the carrot, orange, turmeric root, and lemon juice to a juicer and extract the juice.
5. Stir well and serve immediately.
Serving Size: 1 glass
Nutritional Value: Contains anti-inflammatory properties, vitamin C, and antioxidants.
Cooking Time: 5 minutes

14. Spinach Supreme

Ingredients:
- 2 cups spinach
- 1 cucumber
- 2 green apples
- 1 lemon (juiced)
Instructions:
1. Wash the spinach and cucumber.
2. Chop the cucumber and green apples into small pieces.

3. Add the spinach, cucumber, green apples, and lemon juice to a juicer and extract the juice.

4. Mix well and serve chilled.

Serving Size: 1 glass

Nutritional Value: Rich in vitamins A, C, and K, and antioxidants.

Cooking Time: 5 minutes

15. Papaya Paradise

Ingredients:

- 1 ripe papaya (peeled and seeded)
- 1 orange (peeled)
- 1 lime (juiced)
- 1 tablespoon honey (optional)

Instructions:

1. Chop the papaya into small pieces.

2. Peel the orange and divide it into segments.

3. Juice the lime.

4. Add the papaya, orange segments, lime juice, and honey (if desired) to a blender and blend until smooth.

5. Serve chilled.

Serving Size: 1 glass

Nutritional Value: Contains vitamin C, beta-carotene, and digestive enzymes.
Cooking Time: 5 minutes

16. Ginger Lemonade

Ingredients:
- 2 lemons (juiced)
- 1-inch piece of ginger
- 2 tablespoons honey
- 4 cups water

Instructions:
1. Juice the lemons.
2. Peel the ginger and chop it into small pieces.
3. In a blender, blend the ginger with a little water until smooth.
4. In a pitcher, combine the lemon juice, ginger mixture, honey, and water. Stir well.
5. Serve over ice.

Serving Size: 1 glass
Nutritional Value: Refreshing and aids digestion.
Cooking Time: 10 minutes

17. Mango Madness

Ingredients:
- 2 ripe mangoes (peeled and pitted)
- 1 orange (peeled)
- 1 banana
- 1 cup almond milk

Instructions:
1. Chop the mangoes and banana into chunks.
2. Peel the orange and divide it into segments.
3. Add the mangoes, orange segments, banana, and almond milk to a blender.
4. Blend until smooth and creamy.
5. Serve chilled.

Serving Size: 1 glass
Nutritional Value: Rich in vitamin C, fiber, and potassium.
Preparation Time: 5 minutes

18. Raspberry Refresher

Ingredients:
- 2 cups fresh raspberries
- 1 cup coconut water
- 1 tablespoon lime juice

- 1 tablespoon honey (optional)
Instructions:
1. Wash the raspberries.
2. Add the raspberries, coconut water, lime juice, and honey (if desired) to a blender.
3. Blend until smooth.
4. Serve chilled.
Serving Size: 1 glass
Nutritional Value: High in antioxidants, vitamin C, and electrolytes.
Preparation Time: 5 minutes

19. Carrot Glow

Ingredients:
- 4 large carrots
- 1 orange (peeled)
- 1-inch piece of ginger
- 1 tablespoon honey (optional)
Instructions:
1. Wash and peel the carrots and orange.
2. Chop them into chunks.
3. Peel the ginger.

4. Add the carrot chunks, orange segments, ginger, and honey (if desired) to a juicer or blender.

5. Blend until smooth.

6. Serve chilled.

Serving Size: 1 glass

Nutritional Value: High in beta-carotene, vitamin C, and ginger's anti-inflammatory properties.

Preparation Time: 5 minutes

20. Pomegranate Punch

Ingredients:

- 2 pomegranates
- 1 apple
- 1 lemon (juiced)
- A handful of fresh mint leaves

Instructions:

1. Cut the pomegranates in half and extract the seeds.

2. Wash and chop the apple into chunks.

3. Add the pomegranate seeds, apple chunks, lemon juice, and mint leaves to a juicer or blender.

4. Blend until smooth.

5. Serve chilled.
Serving Size: 1 glass
Nutritional Value: Rich in antioxidants, vitamin C, and mint's digestive properties.
Preparation Time: 5 minutes

21. Citrus Sunrise

Ingredients:
- 2 oranges (peeled)
- 2 grapefruits (peeled)
- 1 lemon (juiced)
- 1 tablespoon honey (optional)

Instructions:
1. Peel the oranges and grapefruits, removing the white pith.
2. Juice the lemon.
3. Add the peeled oranges, peeled grapefruits, lemon juice, and honey (if desired) to a juicer or blender.
4. Blend until smooth.
5. Serve chilled.
Serving Size: 1 glass
Nutritional Value: High in vitamin C, refreshing, and tangy.

Preparation Time: 5 minutes

22. Green Detox

Ingredients:
- 2 cups kale leaves
- 1 cucumber
- 2 green apples
- 1 lemon (juiced)
- 1-inch piece of ginger

Instructions:
1. Wash the kale leaves and cucumber.
2. Chop the cucumber and green apples into chunks.
3. Add the kale leaves, cucumber chunks, green apple chunks, lemon juice, and ginger to a juicer or blender.
4. Blend until smooth.
5. Serve over ice.

Serving Size: 1 glass

Nutritional Value: Detoxifying, rich in vitamins A, C, and K, and aids digestion.

Preparation Time: 5 minutes

23. Minty Melon

Ingredients:
- 2 cups watermelon chunks
- 1 cup honeydew melon chunks
- 1 tablespoon lime juice
- A handful of fresh mint leaves

Instructions:
1. Remove all seeds from the watermelon chunks.
2. Cut the honeydew melon into chunks.
3. Add the watermelon chunks, honeydew melon chunks, lime juice, and fresh mint leaves to a blender.
4. Blend until smooth.
5. Serve chilled.

Serving Size: 1 glass

Nutritional Value: Hydrating, refreshing, and rich in vitamins A, C, and antioxidants.

Preparation Time: 5 minutes

24. Beet Blast

Ingredients:
- 2 beets (peeled and chopped)
- 2 carrots
- 1 apple
- 1-inch piece of ginger
- 1 lemon (juiced)

Instructions:
1. Wash and chop the beets, carrots, and apples into chunks.
2. Peel the ginger.
3. Add the beet chunks, carrot chunks, apple chunks, ginger, and lemon juice to a juicer or blender.
4. Blend until smooth.
5. Serve chilled.

Serving Size: 1 glass

Nutritional Value: Rich in antioxidants, folate, and betalains (beneficial compounds found in beets).

Preparation Time: 5 minutes

25. Berry Beet Bliss

Ingredients:

- 1 cup strawberries
- 1 cup blueberries
- 1 beet (peeled and chopped)
- 1 banana
- 1 cup almond milk

Instructions:

1. Wash the strawberries and blueberries.
2. Peel and chop the beet.
3. Add the strawberries, blueberries, beet chunks, banana, and almond milk to a blender.
4. Blend until smooth and creamy.
5. Serve chilled.

Serving Size: 1 glass

Nutritional Value: Packed with antioxidants, fiber, and vitamins.

Preparation Time: 5 minutes

26. Citrus Ginger Zing

Ingredients:
- 2 oranges (peeled)
- 1 grapefruit (peeled)
- 1 lemon (peeled)
- 1-inch piece of ginger
- 1 tablespoon honey (optional)

Instructions:
1. Peel the oranges, grapefruit, and lemon, removing the white pith.
2. Peel the ginger.
3. Add the peeled oranges, peeled grapefruit, peeled lemon, ginger, and honey (if desired) to a juicer or blender.
4. Blend until smooth.
5. Serve chilled.

Serving Size: 1 glass

Nutritional Value: High in vitamin C, refreshing, and aids digestion.

Preparation Time: 5 minutes

27. Kiwi Lime Cooler

Ingredients:
- 4 kiwis (peeled)
- 1 lime (juiced)
- 1 cup coconut water
- A handful of fresh mint leaves

Instructions:
1. Peel the kiwis and cut them into chunks.
2. Juice the lime.
3. Add the kiwi chunks, lime juice, coconut water, and fresh mint leaves to a blender.
4. Blend until smooth.
5. Serve over ice.

Serving Size: 1 glass

Nutritional Value: Rich in vitamin C, potassium, and refreshing flavors.

Preparation Time: 5 minutes

28. Creamy Avocado Delight

Ingredients:
- 1 ripe avocado (peeled and pitted)
- 1 cup spinach
- 1 green apple

- 1 cucumber
- 1 lemon (juiced)
- A handful of fresh cilantro

Instructions:

1. Wash the spinach and cilantro.
2. Cut the avocado in half, remove the pit, and scoop out the flesh.
3. Chop the green apple and cucumber into chunks.
4. Add the avocado flesh, spinach, green apple chunks, cucumber chunks, lemon juice, and cilantro to a blender.
5. Blend until smooth and creamy.
6. Serve chilled.

Serving Size: 1 glass

Nutritional Value: Packed with healthy fats from avocado, vitamins, and refreshing flavors.

Preparation Time: 5 minutes

29. Ginger Turmeric Elixir

Ingredients:
- 1-inch piece of ginger
- 1-inch piece of turmeric raw or 1 teaspoon turmeric powder
- 2 oranges (peeled)
- 1 carrot
- 1 apple

Instructions:
1. Peel the ginger and turmeric (if using fresh).
2. Juice the oranges.
3. Wash and chop the carrot and apple into chunks.
4. Add the ginger, turmeric, orange juice, carrot chunks, and apple chunks to a juicer or blender.
5. Blend until smooth.
6. Serve chilled.

Serving Size: 1 glass

Nutritional Value: Anti-inflammatory properties from ginger and turmeric, high in vitamin C, and beta-carotene from carrot.

Preparation Time: 5 minutes

30. Creamy Green

Ingredients:
- 2 cups spinach
- 1 cup kale leaves
- 1 cucumber
- 1 green apple
- 1/2 avocado
- 1 tablespoon lemon juice
- 1 cup coconut water

Instructions
1. Wash the spinach, kale, and cucumber.
2. Chop the cucumber and green apple into chunks.
3. Add the spinach, kale leaves, cucumber chunks, green apple chunks, avocado, lemon juice, and coconut water to a juicer or blender.
4. Blend until smooth and creamy.
5. Serve chilled.

Serving Size: 1 glass

Nutritional Value: Packed with vitamins, minerals, fiber, and healthy fats from avocado.

Preparation Time: 5 minutes

Chapter 2: 30 delicious Smoothie Recipes for acne

1. Green Glow Smoothie

Ingredients: Spinach, cucumber, pineapple, coconut water.

Instructions: Blend all ingredients until smooth. Serve chilled.

Nutritional Value: Packed with vitamins A and C, and hydrating properties.

Cooking Time: Approximately 5 minutes.

2. Berry Burst Smoothie

Ingredients: varieties of berries (strawberries, blueberries, raspberries), almond milk, chia seeds.

Instructions: Blend berries and almond milk together. Sprinkle chia seeds on top.

Nutritional Value: High in antioxidants and omega-3 fatty acids.

Cooking Time: Around 3 minutes.

3. Citrus Zing Smoothie

Ingredients: Oranges, lemons, Greek yogurt, honey.
Instructions: Squeeze the juice from oranges and lemons, then blend with yogurt and honey.
Nutritional Value: High in vitamin C and probiotics.
Cooking Time: Approximately 4 minutes.

4. Tropical Delight Smoothie

Ingredients: Mango, banana, coconut milk, turmeric.
Instructions: Blend mango, banana, and coconut milk together. Add a pinch of turmeric for flavor.
Nutritional Value: Provides a dose of vitamin A and anti-inflammatory properties.
Cooking Time: Around 3 minutes.

5. Glow-Getter Smoothie

Ingredients: Carrots, oranges, ginger, almond milk.

Instructions: Blend carrots, oranges, ginger, and almond milk until smooth.

Nutritional Value: Packed with beta-carotene, vitamin C, and anti-inflammatory properties.

Cooking Time: Approximately 5 minutes.

6. Avocado Elixir Smoothie

Ingredients: Avocado, spinach, banana, almond milk.

Instructions: Blend avocado, spinach, banana, and almond milk until creamy.

Nutritional Value: Rich in healthy fats, fiber, and essential vitamins.

Cooking Time: Around 3 minutes.

7. Blueberry Bliss Smoothie

Ingredients: Blueberries, spinach, almond butter, coconut water.

Instructions: Blend blueberries, spinach, almond butter, and coconut water until well combined.

Nutritional Value: Packed with antioxidants, iron, and healthy fats.

Cooking Time: Approximately 4 minutes.

8. Minty Melon Smoothie

Ingredients: Watermelon, cucumber, mint leaves, lime juice.

Instructions: Blend watermelon, cucumber, mint leaves, and lime juice until refreshing.

Nutritional Value: Hydrating, rich in vitamins A and C, and aids in digestion.

Cooking Time: Around 3 minutes.

9. Pineapple Paradise Smoothie

Ingredients: Pineapple, coconut milk, banana, turmeric, honey.

Instructions: Blend pineapple, coconut milk, banana, and a sprinkle of turmeric. Sweeten with honey if desired.

Nutritional Value: Bursting with tropical flavors, vitamin C, and natural anti-inflammatory properties.

Cooking Time: Approximately 4 minutes.

10. Super Berry Blast Smoothie

Ingredients: Acai berries, mixed berries, almond milk, spinach, flaxseeds.

Instructions: Blend acai berries, mixed berries, almond milk, spinach, and a sprinkle of flaxseeds.

Nutritional Value: Packed in antioxidants, fiber, and essential fatty acids.

Cooking Time: Around 3 minutes.

11. Creamy Green Dream Smoothie

Ingredients: Avocado, kale, almond milk, banana, honey.

Instructions: Blend avocado, kale, almond milk, banana, and a drizzle of honey for sweetness.

Nutritional Value: Provides healthy fats, vitamins, and minerals for nourished skin.

Cooking Time: Approximately 4 minutes.

12. Chocolate Bliss Smoothie

Ingredients: Raw cacao powder, almond butter, banana, almond milk, dates.

Instructions: Blend raw cacao powder, almond butter, banana, almond milk, and dates for natural sweetness.

Nutritional Value: Offers antioxidants, magnesium, and a touch of indulgence.

Cooking Time: Around 3 minutes.

13. Golden Sunshine Smoothie

Ingredients: Pineapple, mango, turmeric, ginger, coconut water.

Instructions: Blend pineapple, mango, a sprinkle of turmeric, a hint of ginger, and refreshing coconut water.

Nutritional Value: Brimming with tropical flavors, immune-boosting properties, and anti-inflammatory benefits.

Cooking Time: Approximately 5 minutes.

14. Matcha Magic Smoothie

Ingredients: Matcha powder, banana, almond milk, spinach, honey.

Instructions: Blend matcha powder, banana, almond milk, a handful of spinach, and a touch of honey for sweetness.

Nutritional Value: Provides a gentle energy boost, antioxidants, and a vibrant green hue.

Cooking Time: Around 3 minutes.

15. Protein Powerhouse Smoothie

Ingredients: Greek yogurt, almond butter, banana, spinach, almond milk.

Instructions: Blend Greek yogurt, a dollop of almond butter, banana, a handful of spinach, and creamy almond milk.

Nutritional Value: Offers a protein punch, essential vitamins, and minerals for sustained energy.

Cooking Time: Approximately 4 minutes.

16. Zen Garden Smoothie

Ingredients: Green tea, cucumber, kiwi, honeydew melon, lime juice.

Instructions: Brew a cup of green tea, blend it with sliced cucumber, kiwi, juicy honeydew melon, and a squeeze of lime juice.

Nutritional Value: Refreshing, hydrating, and abundant in antioxidants.

Cooking Time: Around 3 minutes.

17.   Lavender   Dream Smoothie:

Ingredients: Blueberries, lavender buds, almond milk, banana, honey.

Instructions: Blend blueberries, a sprinkle of fragrant lavender buds, creamy almond milk, banana, and a drizzle of honey.

Nutritional Value: Filled with antioxidants, floral aromas, and a touch of sweetness.

Cooking Time: Approximately 4 minutes.

18. Exotic Dragon Smoothie

Ingredients: Dragon fruit, coconut water, pineapple, lime juice, mint leaves.

Instructions: Blend vibrant dragon fruit, hydrating coconut water, juicy pineapple, a squeeze of lime juice, and fresh mint leaves.

Nutritional Value: Bursting with tropical flavors, hydrating properties, and a touch of zing.

Cooking Time: Around 3 minutes.

19. Chia Power Smoothie

Ingredients: Chia seeds, almond milk, mixed berries, spinach, banana.

Instructions: Soak chia seeds in almond milk until gel-like, then blend with mixed berries, spinach, and banana until smooth.

Nutritional Value: Provides a boost of omega-3 fatty acids, fiber, and a medley of vitamins.

Cooking Time: Approximately 4 minutes.

20. Mocha Madness Smoothie:

Ingredients: Cold brew coffee, cacao powder, almond milk, banana, dates.

Instructions: Blend cold brew coffee, a sprinkle of cacao powder, creamy almond milk, banana, and dates for natural sweetness.

Nutritional Value: Offers a delightful balance of coffee and chocolate flavors, antioxidants, and a touch of decadence.
Cooking Time: Around 3 minutes.

21. Enchanted Forest Smoothie

Ingredients: Spinach, kale, green apple, celery, cucumber, lemon juice.
Instructions: Blend together a handful of spinach, kale, a crisp green apple, celery stalks, refreshing cucumber, and a splash of lemon juice.
Nutritional Value: Packed with leafy greens, vitamins, and a burst of zesty flavors.
Cooking Time: Approximately 5 minutes.

22. Cosmic Galaxy Smoothie:

Ingredients: Blackberries, blueberries, purple grapes, coconut milk, acai powder.

Instructions: Blend a mix of blackberries, blueberries, juicy purple grapes, creamy coconut milk, and a sprinkle of acai powder for an otherworldly experience.

Nutritional Value: Filled with antioxidants, anthocyanins, and a touch of cosmic allure.

Cooking Time: Around 3 minutes.

23. Rainbow Bliss Smoothie

Ingredients: Strawberries, mango, pineapple, kiwi, orange juice.

Instructions: Blend a vibrant combination of strawberries, sweet mango, tangy pineapple, zesty kiwi, and a splash of refreshing orange juice.

Nutritional Value: A rainbow of vitamins, tropical flavors, and a burst of sunshine.

Cooking Time: Approximately 4 minutes.

24. Unicorn Sparkle Smoothie

Ingredients: Greek yogurt, raspberries, banana, almond milk, edible glitter (optional).

Instructions: Blend creamy Greek yogurt, plump raspberries, ripe banana, smooth almond milk, and if desired, add a touch of magical edible glitter for that extra sparkle.

Nutritional Value: Creamy, fruity, and a touch of whimsy.

Cooking Time: Around 3 minutes.

25. Mermaid's Delight Smoothie

Ingredients: Spirulina powder, pineapple, coconut milk, banana, lime juice.

Instructions: Blend together the vibrant green spirulina powder, tropical pineapple, creamy coconut milk, ripe banana, and a squeeze of tangy lime juice.

Nutritional Value: Brimming with tropical flavors, antioxidants, and a touch of marine magic.

Cooking Time: Approximately 4 minutes.

26. Phoenix Rising Smoothie

Ingredients: Dragon fruit, mango, papaya, orange juice, cayenne pepper (optional).

Instructions: Blend the fiery dragon fruit, luscious mango, exotic papaya, tangy orange juice, and if you dare, a pinch of fiery cayenne pepper for an invigorating experience.

Nutritional Value: Bursting with tropical goodness, vitamin C, and a hint of spice.

Cooking Time: Around 3 minutes.

27. Fairy Dust Smoothie

Ingredients: Blue spirulina powder, butterfly pea flower tea, coconut water, banana, honey.

Instructions: Blend the mystical blue spirulina powder, infused butterfly pea flower tea, hydrating coconut water, creamy banana, and a drizzle of golden honey for a touch of sweetness.

Nutritional Value: A magical combination of antioxidants, hydration, and whimsical hues.

Cooking Time: Approximately 4 minutes.

28. Centaur's Strength Smoothie

Ingredients: Almond butter, oats, banana, almond milk, maple syrup.

Instructions: Blend the hearty almond butter, nourishing oats, ripe banana, creamy almond milk, and a drizzle of sweet maple syrup for a smoothie that fuels your inner strength.

Nutritional Value: Provides energy, fiber, and a touch of natural sweetness.

Cooking Time: Around 3 minutes.

29. Time Traveler's Elixir Smoothie

Ingredients: Beetroot, strawberries, pomegranate seeds, orange juice, ginger.

Instructions: Blend together the vibrant beetroot, juicy strawberries, tangy pomegranate seeds, zesty orange juice, and a hint of invigorating ginger for a smoothie that transcends time.

Nutritional Value: Packed with antioxidants, vitamins, and a touch of ancient magic.

Preparation Time: Approximately 5 minutes.

30. Galaxy Explorer Smoothie:

Ingredients: Blueberries, blackberries, raspberries, coconut milk, vanilla extract.

Instructions: Blend a constellation of blueberries, blackberries, raspberries, creamy coconut milk, and a dash of fragrant vanilla extract for a smoothie that takes you on a journey through the cosmic expanse.

Nutritional Value: Bursting with antioxidants, natural sweetness, and a taste of the universe.

Preparation Time: Around 3 minutes.

Chapter 3:Bonus

21 tips to reduce acne

1. Hydration:
- Drink plenty of water to keep your skin hydrated and flush out toxins.

2. Balanced Diet:
- Consume a diet rich in fruits, vegetables, and whole foods for essential nutrients.

3. Antioxidant-Rich Foods:
- Include foods high in antioxidants, such as berries, spinach, and green tea.

4. Omega-3 Fatty Acids:
- Incorporate sources of omega-3 fatty acids like fish, flaxseeds, and walnuts.

5. Reduce Dairy Intake:
- Some people find reducing dairy consumption can improve skin condition.

6. Limit Sugar and Processed Foods:

- Minimize the intake of sugary and processed foods, as they can contribute to inflammation.

7. Probiotics:

- Consume probiotic-rich foods like yogurt or consider taking a probiotic supplement for gut health.

8. Regular Exercise:

- Engage in regular physical activity to improve blood circulation and overall health.

9. Stress Management:

- Practice stress-reducing techniques like meditation, yoga, or deep breathing exercises.

10. Adequate Sleep:

- Ensure you get enough quality sleep to support overall well-being.

11. Gentle Cleansing:

   - Use a mild cleanser to wash your face, avoiding harsh products that may irritate the skin.

12. Moisturize:

   - Keep your skin moisturized to prevent excessive dryness.

13. Sun Protection:

   - Use sunscreen to protect your skin from harmful UV rays.

14. Avoid Touching Face:

   - Minimize touching your face to prevent the spread of bacteria.

15. Clean Pillowcases:

   - Change your pillowcases regularly to avoid bacteria buildup.

16. Natural Face Masks:

- Apply natural face masks with ingredients like honey, aloe vera, or clay for skin nourishment.

17. Exfoliation:
- Gently exfoliate your skin to remove dead cells and unclog pores.

18. Tea Tree Oil:
- Consider using tea tree oil, known for its antibacterial properties, as a spot treatment.

19. Non-comedogenic Products:
- Choose skincare and makeup products labeled as non-comedogenic to avoid pore blockage.

20. Avoid Hot Water:
- Wash your face with lukewarm water instead of hot water to prevent skin dryness.

21. Consult a Dermatologist:

- If acne persists, seek advice from a dermatologist for personalized guidance and treatment.

NOTE

These tips focus on maintaining overall skin health, which can contribute to reducing acne. Remember to consult with a healthcare professional for personalized advice based on individual needs and conditions.

Conclusion

As we reach the final pages of "Acne Juicing and Smoothies for Beginners," remember that this isn't just a book about recipes; it's a roadmap to a radiant, confident you. By choosing the right ingredients and embracing the simplicity of juicing and blending, you've embarked on a transformative journey to banish acne from within.

With each sip, you've harnessed the power of nature's goodness, providing your skin with the nutrients it craves. But this isn't the end; it's a new beginning. Your blender is your ally, and these recipes are your secret weapons in the ongoing battle for clearer, healthier skin.

So, here's to you – to the vibrant mornings and soothing evenings, to the refreshing elixirs that became a part of your daily ritual.

Cheers to the journey you've undertaken, the flavors you've savored, and the radiant skin that awaits. As you close this book, carry with you the knowledge that the path to clearer skin is not just a destination but a lifestyle – one sip at a time. Cheers to the beautiful, blemish-free journey ahead!